How I Got to Know
What Caused Cancer
for All These Years

How I Got to Know What Caused Cancer for All These Years

VIC SULTANA

To order additional copies of this book, contact:
Xlibris
1-800-455-039
www.Xlibris.com.au
Orders@Xlibris.com.au
746753

Dedicated to people who are suffering

from cancer and are in pain.

What Is Cancer?

The following information comes from the *National Cancer Institute.*

(https://www.cancer.gov/about-cancer/understanding/what-is-cancer).

Cancer is the name given to a collection of related diseases. In all types of cancer, some of the body's cells begin to divide without stopping and spread into surrounding tissues.

Cancer can start almost anywhere in the human body, which is made up of trillions of cells. Normally, human cells grow and divide to form new cells as the body needs them. When cells grow old or become damaged, they die, and new cells take their place.

When cancer develops, however, this orderly process breaks down. As cells become more and more abnormal, old or damaged cells survive when they should die, and new cells form when they are not needed. These extra cells can divide without stopping and may form growths called tumours.

Many cancers form solid tumours, which are masses of tissue. Cancers of the blood, such as leukemias, generally do not form solid tumours.

Cancerous tumours are malignant, which means they can spread into, or invade, nearby tissues. In addition, as these tumours grow, some cancer cells can break off and travel to distant places in the body through the blood or the lymph system and form new tumours far from the original tumour.

Unlike malignant tumours, benign tumours do not spread into, or invade, nearby tissues. Benign tumours can sometimes be quite large, however. When removed, they usually don't grow back, whereas malignant tumours sometimes do. Unlike most benign tumours elsewhere in the body, benign brain tumours can be life threatening.

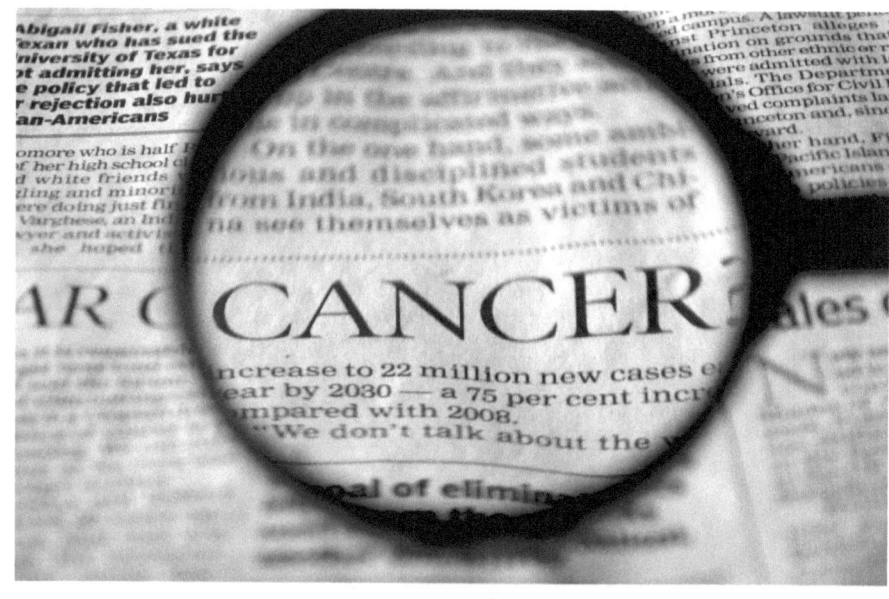

This is the start of my story...

My name is Vic Sultana. I was born in Xaghra Gozo, Malta, in August 1945, just after the end of the Second World War. My parents had fifteen kids, and I was number twelve. Nine are still alive—five brothers and four sisters. The older brothers came to Australia one by one after the war, and that left my mother with four sisters and me. I was only eight or nine years old when I arrived in Australia, and three sisters were younger than me.

That was a drama. We came by ship, and it took three months because there was war at the Suez Canal. The first stop was Cape Town and the second was

Bombay, I think. There were some other ports, but I can't remember them; it was a long time ago. I recall the first stop in Australia was Fremantle, and after that was Melbourne. For the ship, it was the end of the journey; it was supposed to go to Sydney.

My older brother came down for us in a tipper truck from Sydney. Believe me, it was a trip that I will never forget. We had a big wooden box with us. After fifteen hours, we arrived in Sydney. To me, it was an eyesore because I had never seen anything like this before. We never saw any water along the way—for fifteen hours. I thought, *Where are we? The trees are so big and tall. We are in a different world.* We had never seen trains, big cars, and so on.

My older brother was married, and his wife's parents had a poultry farm. He had two tipper trucks. I was working in the farm before and after school like a slave, but that was people did in those days. I went to school at Patrician Brothers in Fairfield, New South Wales, for form 4 class to 3 year.

I left school at the age of fifteen and then worked in a factory for a few months. It was too far to travel, so I found a job in Smithfield, which was close to home. I had an apprenticeship with a cabinetmaker. Eventually Tom, the man who taught me, did not want to teach me anymore because I was Maltese; he was a Pommy anyway. The boss came and said that he was too old to teach anybody. He then asked, "Would you mind going out in the yard and working as a machinist?" I was only fifteen years old, but I said yes.

The factory had a big bin for the shavings. When it was full of shavings, I told my brother to bring the truck and leave it there. After work, I climbed in the bin, pushed down the shavings, and took the truck back to the farm. That went on for a few months.

When I got to the right age, I got a truck licence, and that was the start of my career. I drove tipper trucks all my life.

I got married in 1967, when I was xxx years old. As the years went by, I got sicker and sicker, and I couldn't find anything wrong with me. Nothing showed on tests, but I was in pain, and as years went by, the pain got worse.

It started thirty-five or more years ago with a lot of headaches that lasted for several days. The only way to stop them was to go to the hospital and get an injection to put me to sleep. That went on for years. I would go to hospitals for two weeks and have all the examinations and tests, but nothing would show up. Then in another month or so, I would get another attack, and it would be the same story all over again. It went on for years. I could not have a drink of beer or any other sort of alcohol; it would give me a headache, and I would suffer for a long time. No one could help me, so for that reason, I never drank.

As the years went on, my body started to blow up, bit by bit. I could not work out what was doing it. I would go to the doctors, and the first thing they'd say was, "You have to watch your diet and go for walks to lose that weight."

I responded, "But I'm in pain."

"Well, there is nothing wrong with you," the doctor said. "I can't give you anything, because I can't find anything wrong. Go home and take some Panadol every four hours."

I went home, still in pain, and didn't know what to do. For years, I was in and out of hospitals.

The doctors always said, "We can't find anything wrong. Go home with the pain and try to live with it. You have to adapt to the pain for the rest of your life."

For years, I had pain in my stomach, my head, my bones, my ears, and my gastric system. I saw doctors and visited hospitals, spending days in hospitals getting all the exams, X-rays, and more. You name the test, and I had it, but still they could not find anything. So back home I went, and back to work.

When I was still in pain, sometimes it got so bad that tears came from my eyes. I thought, *God, there must be something that they can do. Surely.* Day after day, the pain changed from one place in the body to another. It got very nasty.

One year, we decided to move from Sydney to Tasmania because of our son. It's a long story! We moved to a place called St. Helens. I was still suffering with headaches and was in bed for two to three days, crying with headaches. This went on for months and years, and it included pain in my stomach and my ears. I would go to the GP and say that I was in pain, so they took me to hospital. Here we went again with all the tests—blood tests, X-rays, MRIs—but they found nothing. I had a few operations during this time. One of them was an open-heart surgery. I had others, but I won't go into all the details.

After two or three years, my headaches weren't so bad, but I could not work out what was going on. After that, the pain started coming back, and it was very severe. I had awful headaches and severe pain in my stomach. I went back to the doctors. Oh, by the way, we had no family doctors for about ten years; they came for maybe five weeks and then went back where they had come from, so that made it very bad for everyone here in St. Helens, especially for those who were sick like me. There were lots of aged people here in those days. We were given a lot of wrong medications, and so on.

Were we started again with the same problem. I went to see doctors about my pain and told them about it. They said, "Here are some antibiotics. Take this, and good luck."

But the antibiotics didn't work, so I went back to hospital and had operations for hernias. The first operation was a drama. Two days after the operation, it started to swell up like a balloon. I had an ultrasound, and they found nothing to worry about. "It's just a little bit of water."

The next day I wanted to go home, and they let me go! Off to home we went.

In Kings Meadows two days later, the swelling started to rise, and it was like a balloon. That night, it burst open. The hole was bigger than a fifty-cent piece. I nearly died when I saw it. Back to the hospital we went.

They said it was infected but did nothing to it. They said, "Just keep cleaning it, and it will close by itself."

Two or three weeks later, I had to have an operation. I was in and out of hospitals and saw doctors and specialists like it was fashionable, but I was in pain all the time. My ears never stopped ringing for forty years, with no relief. Every time I had holidays, I ended up in hospital. They were my holidays all my life.

My eyes were always watering, I was sneezing all the same time, and I was putting on weight even though I was not eating rubbish food. I kept saying, "What is wrong with me?"

My life was changing. Between the headaches and the bloating, when I went to bed at night, I lay down and cried, "What is happening to my life, God? What am I doing wrong? Please help me, and guide me to get my life back." I prayed every night with tears in my eyes.

We had a pet dog named Susie, and she was one off. To make the story short, she ended up getting cancer, so we took her to the vet to remove it. That went good, but as time passed, Susie started to blow up for no reason. She was so active and a goer, but she started to slow down a lot.

Again, at night with tears in my eyes, I prayed, "Help me, God. I don't know what to do anymore. Please help me."

A few months later, that lump on Susie came back. "Oh, God, it came back. No! It can't be happening. The air here is so pure. It can't be happening." We went back to the vet to have it removed, and it cost an arm and a leg every time we went to that blessed vet because he was the only one here. Back home we went, and as time went by, Susie got fatter for no reason and ended up with brain tumor, which we did not realize that she had. We lost her in June 2009, and that broke my heart. For weeks I was lost without her, and I kept saying to myself, "Why her, God?" But there was more to this.

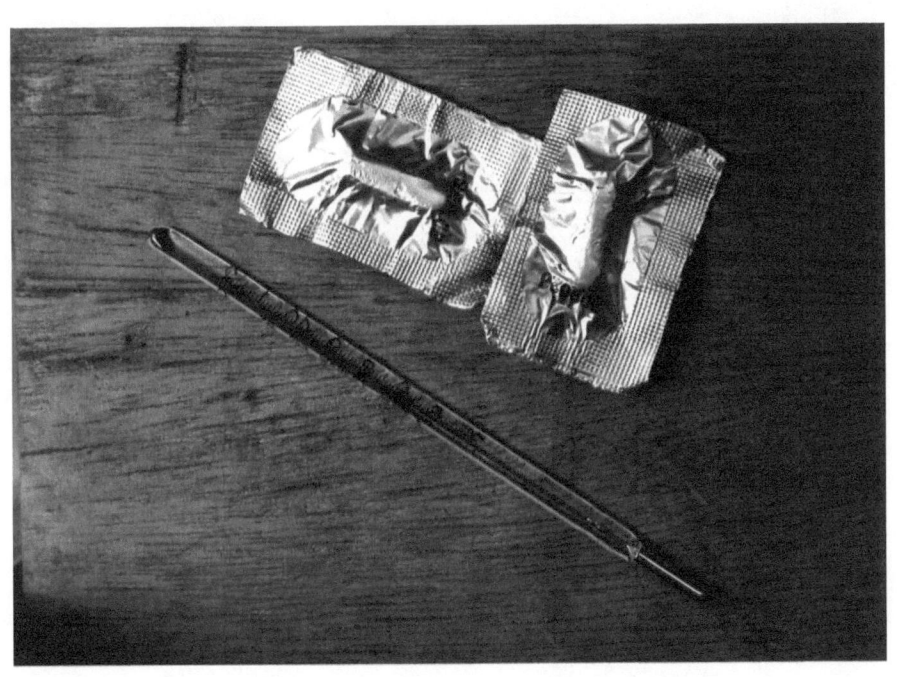

As time went by, things were getting worse for me day by day. After a few years, we had found another two pets, Max and Molly. The owner of them wanted to give them away because he could not keep them due to his job. I rang the fellow up and said that I was interested; we had a bit of land that would be nice for them. He told us that he would bring them the following Sunday. We could not wait for that Sunday to come.

The day arrived, and out of the car they came, running and nervous because they did not know what was happening. I had not met the owner before, and I did not know what to say to him, but I shook hands with him, and we started talking about Max and Molly. They were courageous, and I could not keep my eyes off of them. The owner said, "They are all yours, but you have to promise me something."

I said, "Yes, what is it?" I didn't know what to think.

"If you decide to keep them, then you will never separate them. Promise me that."

We shook hands, and I said that would never happen while I was still alive. I fell in love with them the minute I saw them.

It took a good while till they adjusted to us, but we have spoiled them rotten. As time went by, they started to get runny eyes, and they sneezed too. Molly started to blow up too, and she was not eating much either. It was the same problem that was happening to us: sore eyes, sneezing, bloating. At night I lay in bed, tears running down eyes. "God, please help me to find what is going on in our house. I really don't know what to do anymore."

One day in October 2014, my wife was doing voluntary at Media Park and at the church, so she was out all day. I was sitting on the toilet, and I was sneezing. At the same time, Max came in and he was sneezing too.

I thought there must be something in this house that was doing this to us. This was when I started to look for what was causing this. I pulled everything out of the cupboard, and I found six packets. It was so strong that when I opened the door, it threw me back. "Wow," I said to Max. We took them out of the house, plus all the other stuff, and opened windows for fresh air to come in. When my wife came back, she said, "What's this? No wonder we are all dying, with all these fumes. Fancy having packets in the house!" They stung that much, and they were there for over eight years. We were going along and arguing about this and that, and we ended up finding one of those packets in every room for crying out loud. Wow, no wonder we were all sick! We were very lucky that we did not end up with cancer.

As time went by, I was trying to clear the air in the house, but Max and Molly were vomiting a lot. We thought it was the food, and there is a lot more to go with this.

As time went by, she got more upset over what I had found, so the packets went in the garbage bin. The headaches were slowing down, and our eyes were watering less. Our pets where breathing better for a while, and their eyes were clearer. My headaches were less often, and my aching body was saying thanks. But again, there was a lot more to go with this.

As we go back, I was getting a lot cramps in my body, so I thought it was one of my nerves. I made an appointment with chiropractor. I was in agony, so I went to the chiropractor and told him what was happening, adding that I was getting a lot of cramps at night and was worried that I might get blockage.

He said to me, "Vic, it's not your nerves giving the cramps to you. It's one of your tablets that's doing that to you." He did what he had to do to my body, and I thanked him for it, and for the information that he gave me. When I got home, we went through my tablets. One of the tablets was called Lipitor. I went down the doctors— here we went again.

I told him about the tablet and he said, "Oh, yes, they have some potential to do that if you take them for a long time." He gave me another tablet that worked, thank God.

For my wife, it got to her in her brain, and she developed a second personality. The more she inhaled it, the worse she got, and every morning she blew up for no reason. When she got out of the house and did something in the garden, outside in the fresh air, she would come back to normal. The longer she stayed in the house and smelled that shit, the worse she got, but only against me. I could not work that out, because if she was with someone else, butter would not melt in her mouth!

As time went by, she got worse, and I could not control her. No one knew what was going on. I talked to a doctor about it, and he said all women did that. I said that the fumes that we were smelling caused it. He started laughing like I was mad. It was not in their medical books, so they didn't want to know about it.

Where we were, on top of the hill, she would scream and become vicious and cranky. While that was going on, she was in a rage. Depending on how long she stayed in the house, it could go for a few hours or even five days. I got her to take away that stuff, with a lot of difficulty and screaming that I was mad and crazy. After arguing and carrying for weeks on end, I lost it. As I removed the packets bit by bit, she started to come back to what she was, but it had affected her brain. No one knows what I have been through, but that's domestic.

As she was taking one packet away, she was bringing some other shit in the house. I started to get headaches real bad again. What the hell was going on here? Molly's and Max's eyes started to water, so I went to my wife again. "You must have something back in the house, for us to get like this again."

Well, World War Three hit. She said, "You are mad. There is nothing here!" In the meantime, she was smelling it herself, and she became like she was before.

In the meantime, I was back to the doctors for pain. They gave me some strong tablets to take. I tried to get rid of the stuff she bought home, but she hid it in the house, and that made it worse. Sometimes I found it and destroyed it. The story went on; if I keep going, there would not be not enough pages to finish the story.

As we came down, I kept saying to her, "Please understand that we are allergic to that shit, not only me but all of us. Can you understand that? Even you! It gets in your brain, and you do things that you don't know that you are doing. Till it gets out of your system, you give me hell and tell people that I'm mad and have lost it."

After many months, the message got through to her. That shit was not good for us, so got rid of it and started to become normal. After a lot of fresh air, it was a pleasure to sit in our house and not breathe that shit. I thanked her for understanding and keeping our house away from that shit. But in her mind I was still crazy. Our pets' eyes were wonderful, but the shit took a long time to get out of our systems.

When I found out about the shit that had caused all the pain and suffering for many years, after a while, my headaches went away, my eyes stopped being sore and watering, my aching body started to slow down, and my bloating stopped.

I went to the doctor and told him what was wrong with me, adding that I couldn't smell that shit anymore. He sort of laughed about it. I said to him, "What's so funny? I have been smelling that shit for the past forty-five years, and I have found out what cause it. You are telling me that I'm mad!" I had to shake my head. "Would you give me something for the pain?" He would not believe what I told him, so after a while I changed doctors.

I told the new doctor about what I'd said to other one, and he said to me, "There is no such a thing about the smell you're smelling." I asked for more pain killers, and he gave me some more. What was I going to do? Who was I going to see? No one wanted to know about it because it was not in their books. They really didn't want to talk about it. This was in October 2014, and I thought there must be someone I could talk to.

The system I had was the same system of cancer, and believe me, trying to explain to the doctors was very hard. I had tried so hard to try to help people, to find someone and explain what caused it. It was a bloody drama, believe you me.

I rang all the television stations to see if I could talk to someone about it, and they asked me the same question: what was it about? I said it was about cancer.

One of the stations said to me, "I'll send a TV crew next week for you." The other wanted something in writing.

I told them, "Would you please listen to what I have to say? It will stop a lot of people from suffering pain and dying." It went in one ear and out the other. I thought, *Lord, there has to be someone to hear me out. What have people got to lose?*

I rang the newspapers, and when they asked me what it was about, I'd say cancer. They reacted like I was a criminal! "Would you please hear me out?" I'd say before they hung up. "A lot of people are suffering with pain and dying."

I'll have someone get back to you," they said, and that was the last time I heard from them. They should be shot for not listening. God help them. What would it have taken to simply listen?

In the meantime, back to the doctor I went, still in pain. I was surviving from day to day, and the tablets I took kept the pain down a bit. The doctor gave me painkillers for the fourth time with him. I asked him to give me some chemo. He asked why. "All the tablets I have had in the past have done nothing. Really, it made me worse, and I always have an upset stomach from all the tablets." I was taking nearly eighteen tablets a day, and when I was taking them, I always had an upset stomach. All time I felt that I wanted to chuck, and I had cramps at night. The more tablets I took, the worse my body got.

I went to the doctors and explained my pain to him. He said, "Well, we'd better change the tablets." Some of the tablets were not on the prescriptions, they were costly. They still couldn't work it out what's wrong with me, and it went on for so long. It was a wonder that I was still alive given what I had been through.

I used tablets to go to sleep, and the more tablets I took, the worse I got. The same thing happened to my wife and our pets. It hit my wife in a different way. She was getting fat too and didn't know why, and we didn't stop working. It affected her brain, and she became very aggressive and domineering, with a very venom tongue. Whatever she said, whether it was right or wrong, that was the way it went. She would argue for the sake of it, till she got it off her chest. Then we'd go outside in the fresh air, and she'd come back to normal. There is more to explain about it and how it went, but that would be another long story to see what the smell had caused.

In the end, I have started to be my own doctor, mixing some of the tables they gave me in the past to survive. That started in 2014. I have found what caused the smell. It took me nearly eighteen months to get through to my wife, and I was glad that did.

Since that day in 2014, I've cleared the air in the house and all around us. My headaches have disappeared, my eyes have stopped watering, and my pains have eased. I have stopped more than half of my tablets, but the smell got into my body so much that it's still giving me hell as I get it out of my body.

I went to the GP and told him what I was experiencing. He looked at me and laughed about it!

Back home, I went to my shed and mucked around with some timber to pass the day. No matter what I took for my pain, nothing seemed to work. As time went by, I was putting together what I had been through, and how cancer was happening in my body. I knew exactly what it did and how it grew.

I can stop it from growing, but that depends on the person who is suffering. Let me help you too. There's nothing to lose. I can even help people with migraines and other sicknesses.

At the last doctor that I saw, I begged him to give me some chemo. He looked at me and said, "But what for?"

I told him again and again that the tablets and antibiotics, and all the other medicines, did not work for me. It didn't matter what doses I took; they did not help me. The only chance I had left was chemo. I said, "Why don't you want to give chemo? Will it kill me?"

He said, "No, it won't kill you, but it won't make you better than you are now, with all the pain that you have." He thought about it for a while. "First I want you to go have X-rays for your bowels, and then we will see what's going on."

The following week, he said to me that I had some stool caught on my left side, and at the end of day, he ended up giving me some chemo. "But you only to take two tablets a week."

I'm on that now, and it's a low dose, but you would not believe what it's done so far. The smell and the disease that I had in my body had been there for a long time, so it was not going to come out in one day. (More to explain about this too.)

If, there is someone out who wants to hear me out, I'm sure it will help the damned thing from growing any further. Regarding my headaches, chemo has stopped them. I can't see why it wouldn't help you too.

It goes into the body in different ways, and not all bodies are the same. It affects the weakest point of origin, whether it's a baby or an adult. Every time I hear "cancer," my body goes cold. I know that I can help, but I say, "God, don't let people suffer, please." How was I going to go out there and tell them that I could help? Some people may be too far gone.

But even if I can help one out of five or ten, that would give an idea, for the scientists to go on! It would be a breakthrough. I think it would be better to go overseas. They might listen more. I really don't know anymore. There is no money involved with this whatsoever, so don't think it is about money, because it's not! This is to help you, trying to stop it from the suffering that you are going true.

It will help all kinds with cancer, and it'll help the eyes from burning or running, arthritis, and migraines.

I need to prove it first and find someone to trust me. It will be good to find a good listener, like a professor or scientist, whom I can trust and who can help me out and get the message out there.

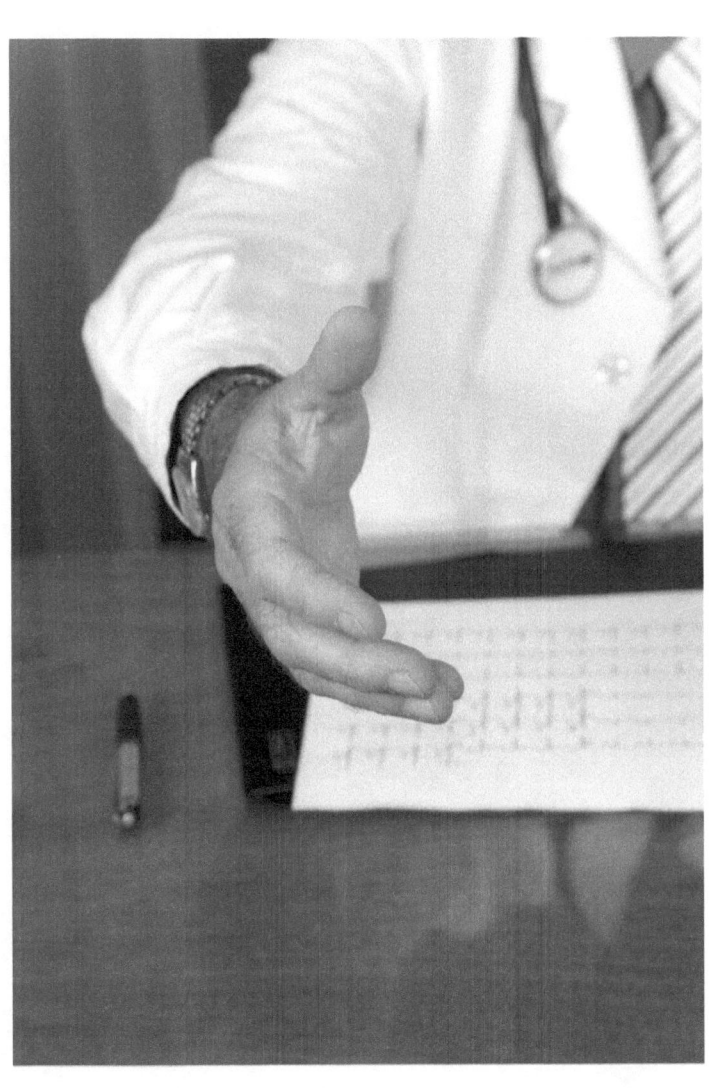

I'm seventy years old and retired. I want to get this message out before I die. I have found the cause of cancer, and I would like to see a big church getting built or a big cathedral, and where I am sitting, they can place an altar!

But how am I going to go about this? If the book goes out, people are going to go mad. All I'm after is one person to tell me how I'm going to go about it. I really know what has caused it, but I'm frightened because I can see what's going to happen. Please help me go about it! I'm really afraid, but I want to get this out, and the sooner the better. There are people suffering and dying, but I'm afraid about how to go about it.

If there are two scientists and professors who can listen and understand, I can explain it to them first. I can go on forever, but let's see if anyone can help me, in order to help others.

If you can help, I can only say from my heart, thank you so much!